DR. BARBARA GREEN SMOOTHIES FOR CANCER

Discover Dr. Barbara's powerful green smoothies-step-by-guide to cancer cure using simple, nutrient-rich recipes

Felipe Carmen

Table of Contents

COPYRIGHT © 2023

CHAPTER ONE

Introduction to Dr. Barbara's Healing Method: Understanding the Principles of Natural Healing and Cancer Remission

Dr. Barbara's Healing Method is a holistic approach to natural healing and cancer remission developed by Dr. Barbara, a renowned integrative medicine practitioner with decades of experience in the field. This method encompasses a comprehensive understanding of the body's innate healing abilities and seeks to empower individuals to take control of their health and well-being through a combination of lifestyle changes, nutritional interventions, mind-body techniques, and alternative therapies.

At the core of Dr. Barbara's Healing Method lies the principle that the body has an inherent ability to heal itself when provided with the right conditions and support. Unlike conventional medicine, which often focuses solely on treating symptoms and managing diseases with pharmaceutical interventions, this approach addresses the root causes of illness and promotes holistic healing on physical, mental, emotional, and spiritual levels.

Understanding the Principles of Natural Healing

Natural healing is based on the belief that the body possesses its own intelligence and mechanisms for self-repair and regeneration. This principle is rooted in the concept of vitalism, which views life as more than just the sum of its chemical and biological components but as an expression of a vital force or energy that animates living organisms.

According to natural healing principles, health is not merely the absence of disease but a state of balance and harmony within the body, mind, and spirit. When this balance is disrupted due to various factors such as poor diet, stress, environmental toxins, or emotional trauma, it can manifest as illness or disease.

The goal of natural healing is to restore this balance by removing obstacles to health and supporting the body's inherent healing mechanisms. This may involve dietary and lifestyle modifications, detoxification, stress reduction techniques, supplementation with vitamins and minerals, herbal medicine, acupuncture, energy healing, and other alternative therapies.

Cancer Remission: A Holistic Approach

Cancer remission refers to the partial or complete disappearance of cancerous cells and tumors in response to treatment. While conventional cancer treatments such as surgery, chemotherapy, and radiation therapy can be effective in eliminating cancer cells, they often come with significant side effects and may not address the underlying causes of the disease.

Dr. Barbara's Healing Method takes a holistic approach to cancer remission by addressing not only the physical aspects of the disease but also the mental, emotional, and spiritual factors that may contribute to its development and progression. This approach recognizes that cancer is a multifactorial disease influenced by genetics, lifestyle choices, environmental factors, emotional stress, and unresolved trauma.

In addition to conventional cancer treatments, Dr. Barbara's Healing Method may incorporate a variety of complementary and alternative therapies to support the body's natural ability to heal and enhance the effectiveness of treatment. These may include nutritional therapy, detoxification protocols, immune support, mind-body techniques such as meditation and visualization, energy healing modalities like Reiki or Qi Gong, and psychospiritual counseling.

Key Principles of Dr. Barbara's Healing Method

1. **Nutritional Therapy:** A cornerstone of Dr. Barbara's Healing Method is the emphasis on whole foods nutrition tailored to individual needs. This may include a plant-based diet rich in fruits, vegetables, whole grains, nuts, and seeds, as well as organic, locally sourced, and minimally processed foods.

Nutritional supplements may also be recommended to address specific deficiencies and support immune function.

2. **Detoxification:** The body's ability to eliminate toxins is crucial for optimal health and cancer prevention. Dr. Barbara's Healing Method may incorporate various detoxification protocols such as fasting, juicing, colon cleansing, sauna therapy, and lymphatic drainage to support the body's natural detoxification pathways and enhance the elimination of harmful substances.

3. **Stress Reduction:** Chronic stress weakens the immune system and contributes to inflammation, which can promote the growth and spread of cancer cells. Mind-body techniques such as meditation, deep breathing, yoga, tai chi, and biofeedback are integral components of Dr. Barbara's Healing Method for reducing stress, promoting relaxation, and restoring balance to the nervous system.

4. **Emotional Healing:** Unresolved emotional issues and trauma can create energetic blockages in the body and compromise its ability to heal. Dr. Barbara's Healing Method may include psychotherapy, counseling, emotional release techniques, and energy psychology modalities such as Emotional Freedom Techniques (EFT) or EMDR (Eye Movement Desensitization and Reprocessing) to address emotional imbalances and support psychological healing.

5. **Spiritual Connection:** Cultivating a sense of purpose, meaning, and spiritual connection can provide profound support and healing during the cancer journey. Practices such as prayer, meditation, mindfulness, journaling, and connecting with nature are encouraged as ways to tap into the deeper dimensions of healing and foster a sense of inner peace, resilience, and hope.

Conclusion

Dr. Barbara's Healing Method offers a comprehensive and integrative approach to natural healing and cancer remission that addresses the physical, mental, emotional, and spiritual aspects of health and well-being. By empowering individuals to take an active role in their healing journey and addressing the underlying causes of illness, this method holds the promise of not only treating cancer but also restoring health, vitality, and wholeness on all levels of being.

CHAPTER TWO

The Role of Nutrition in Cancer Treatment: Exploring How Green Smoothies Can Support the Body's Healing Processes

Nutrition plays a vital role in cancer treatment, offering a powerful tool for supporting the body's healing processes and enhancing the effectiveness of conventional therapies. Among the myriad of nutritional interventions available, green smoothies have gained popularity for their nutrient-rich composition and potential health benefits. In this exploration, we delve into the role of nutrition in cancer treatment, focusing specifically on how green smoothies can contribute to the body's healing journey.

Understanding the Importance of Nutrition in Cancer Treatment

Nutrition is a cornerstone of cancer treatment, providing essential nutrients that support immune function, promote tissue repair, and help mitigate the side effects of therapy. Cancer and its treatments can place significant demands on the body, leading to nutritional deficiencies, weight loss, muscle wasting, and compromised immune function. Therefore, optimizing nutritional intake is crucial for maintaining strength, vitality, and overall well-being during cancer treatment.

A well-balanced diet rich in fruits, vegetables, whole grains, lean proteins, and healthy fats provides the essential nutrients needed to support the body's healing processes and enhance treatment outcomes. These nutrients include vitamins, minerals, antioxidants, phytonutrients, fiber, and omega-3 fatty acids, all of which play unique roles in promoting health and fighting disease.

The Nutritional Benefits of Green Smoothies

Green smoothies are a convenient and delicious way to incorporate a variety of nutrient-dense foods into the diet, particularly leafy green vegetables, fruits, and other healthful ingredients. The primary components of green smoothies typically include leafy greens such as spinach, kale, Swiss chard, or collard greens, combined with fruits like bananas, berries, apples, or pineapple, and liquid such as water, coconut water, or almond milk.

The nutritional benefits of green smoothies stem from their rich array of vitamins, minerals, antioxidants, and phytonutrients. Leafy greens are particularly nutrient-dense, containing vitamins A, C, K, and folate, as well as minerals like calcium, magnesium, and potassium. These nutrients support immune function, bone health, cardiovascular health, and cellular repair mechanisms, all of which are essential during cancer treatment.

Fruits contribute natural sweetness, flavor, and additional nutrients to green smoothies, including vitamin C, fiber, and various antioxidants such as flavonoids and polyphenols. Berries, in particular, are known for their high antioxidant content, which helps combat oxidative stress and inflammation, both of which play key roles in cancer development and progression.

How Green Smoothies Support the Body's Healing Processes

Green smoothies offer several ways in which they can support the body's healing processes during cancer treatment:

1. **Nutrient Density:** Green smoothies provide a concentrated source of essential nutrients in an easily digestible and absorbable form. This is particularly beneficial for individuals experiencing appetite loss, nausea, or difficulty chewing and swallowing due to cancer treatment side effects.

2. **Hydration:** Maintaining adequate hydration is essential for overall health and well-being, especially during cancer treatment. Green smoothies, which typically contain water or other hydrating liquids, can help keep the body well-hydrated and support proper cellular function, detoxification, and waste elimination.

3. **Immune Support:** The vitamins, minerals, antioxidants, and phytonutrients found in green smoothies help bolster immune function and enhance the body's ability to fight infections, inflammation, and disease. A strong immune

system is essential for combating cancer and supporting recovery from treatment-related side effects.

4. **Digestive Health:** The fiber content of green smoothies supports digestive health by promoting regularity, preventing constipation, and nourishing beneficial gut bacteria. A healthy digestive system is essential for nutrient absorption, detoxification, and overall well-being.

5. **Antioxidant Protection:** Green smoothies are rich in antioxidants, which help neutralize harmful free radicals and protect cells from oxidative damage. This is particularly important during cancer treatment, as oxidative stress is implicated in cancer development, treatment resistance, and tissue damage.

Incorporating Green Smoothies into Cancer Treatment

Integrating green smoothies into a cancer treatment regimen can be a simple and enjoyable way to enhance nutritional intake and support the body's healing processes. However, it's essential to customize smoothie recipes to individual preferences, dietary restrictions, and treatment-related side effects. For example, individuals undergoing chemotherapy may need to avoid certain fruits or ingredients that exacerbate nausea or taste alterations.

Consulting with a registered dietitian or nutritionist who specializes in oncology can provide personalized guidance and recommendations for incorporating green smoothies and other nutritious foods into a cancer treatment plan. Additionally, experimenting with different ingredients, flavors, and textures can help make green smoothies more palatable and enjoyable for individuals undergoing cancer treatment.

In conclusion, nutrition plays a crucial role in cancer treatment, offering numerous benefits for supporting the body's healing processes and enhancing treatment outcomes. Green smoothies, with their nutrient-rich composition and potential health benefits, can be a valuable addition to a cancer treatment regimen, providing essential nutrients, hydration, immune support, digestive health, and antioxidant protection. By incorporating green smoothies and other nutritious foods into their diet, individuals undergoing cancer treatment can nourish their bodies, promote healing, and improve their overall quality of life.

CHAPTER THREE

Dr. Barbara's Philosophy on Herbal Nutrition: Embracing Plant-Based Healing for Cancer Recovery

Dr. Barbara, a leading figure in integrative medicine and holistic health, advocates for a philosophy of herbal nutrition centered around embracing plant-based healing as a cornerstone of cancer recovery. With a deep understanding of the therapeutic potential of herbs and botanicals, Dr. Barbara emphasizes the importance of harnessing the healing power of nature to support the body's innate ability to heal and overcome illness. In this exploration, we delve into Dr. Barbara's philosophy on herbal nutrition and its role in promoting cancer recovery.

The Healing Power of Plants

Plants have been used for thousands of years by traditional healing systems around the world for their medicinal properties and therapeutic benefits. Herbal medicine, also known as botanical medicine or phytotherapy, relies on the use of plants and plant extracts to prevent and treat various health conditions, including cancer.

Herbs contain a diverse array of bioactive compounds, including vitamins, minerals, antioxidants, phytonutrients, essential oils, and other phytochemicals, which exert a wide range of biological effects in the body. These compounds have been shown to possess anti-inflammatory, antioxidant, immune-modulating, anti-proliferative, and apoptotic properties, making them valuable allies in the fight against cancer.

Herbal Nutrition in Cancer Recovery

Dr. Barbara's philosophy on herbal nutrition revolves around the belief that the body has an innate ability to heal itself when provided with the right nutrients and support. Herbal nutrition emphasizes the consumption of nutrient-dense herbs and botanicals as a means of nourishing the body, boosting immune function, reducing inflammation, and supporting overall health and well-being.

In the context of cancer recovery, herbal nutrition plays a multifaceted role in supporting the body's healing processes:

1. **Immune Support:** Many herbs possess immune-enhancing properties, helping to strengthen the body's natural defense mechanisms and improve immune function. Herbs such as echinacea, astragalus, medicinal mushrooms (such as reishi, shiitake, and maitake), and Andrographis paniculata are known for their immune-modulating effects, which can be particularly beneficial for individuals undergoing cancer treatment.

2. **Anti-Inflammatory Action:** Chronic inflammation is a hallmark of cancer and contributes to tumor growth,

progression, and treatment resistance. Herbal remedies with anti-inflammatory properties, such as turmeric, ginger, boswellia, and green tea, help reduce inflammation and support tissue healing and repair.

3. **Antioxidant Protection:** Oxidative stress, resulting from an imbalance between free radicals and antioxidants in the body, is implicated in cancer development and progression. Herbs rich in antioxidants, such as green tea, grapeseed extract, bilberry, and rosemary, help neutralize free radicals and protect cells from oxidative damage.

4. **Detoxification Support:** Supporting the body's natural detoxification pathways is essential for eliminating toxins, metabolic waste products, and environmental pollutants that may contribute to cancer risk and progression. Herbs like milk thistle, dandelion root, burdock root, and cilantro support liver function and enhance detoxification processes.

5. **Stress Reduction:** Chronic stress weakens the immune system and exacerbates inflammation, making it detrimental to overall health and well-being, including cancer recovery. Adaptogenic herbs such as ashwagandha, holy basil, rhodiola, and licorice root help modulate the body's stress response and promote resilience to stressors.

Integrating Herbal Nutrition into Cancer Recovery

Integrating herbal nutrition into a cancer recovery plan involves personalized guidance and recommendations tailored to individual needs, preferences, and health goals. Dr. Barbara emphasizes the importance of consulting with a qualified healthcare practitioner, such as a naturopathic doctor, herbalist, or integrative oncologist, who can provide individualized support and guidance based on a comprehensive assessment of each patient's health status, medical history, and treatment plan.

When incorporating herbal nutrition into cancer recovery, it's essential to prioritize safety, quality, and efficacy. Choosing high-quality, organic herbs from reputable sources and avoiding potential interactions with medications or treatments are important considerations. Additionally, starting with low doses and gradually increasing as tolerated can help minimize adverse reactions and optimize therapeutic benefits.

In conclusion, Dr. Barbara's philosophy on herbal nutrition underscores the importance of embracing plant-based healing as a fundamental aspect of cancer recovery. By harnessing the therapeutic potential of herbs and botanicals, individuals undergoing cancer treatment can nourish their bodies, support immune function, reduce inflammation, enhance detoxification, and promote overall health and well-being. Through personalized guidance and a holistic approach to care, herbal nutrition offers a valuable adjunctive therapy in the journey towards healing and wellness.

CHAPTER FOUR

Understanding Cancer: Insights into the Disease Process and Lifestyle Factors that Influence Cancer Development

Cancer is a complex and multifaceted disease characterized by the uncontrolled growth and spread of abnormal cells in the body. It encompasses a diverse range of conditions that can affect virtually any organ or tissue and is influenced by a combination of genetic, environmental, and lifestyle factors. In this exploration, we delve into the disease process of cancer and examine the lifestyle factors that play a critical role in its development.

The Disease Process of Cancer

Cancer arises from the accumulation of genetic mutations and alterations that disrupt the normal regulatory mechanisms controlling cell growth, proliferation, and death. These mutations can occur spontaneously or be induced by various factors, including exposure to carcinogens, genetic predisposition, chronic inflammation, and immune dysfunction.

The hallmark of cancer is uncontrolled cell growth, fueled by the activation of oncogenes (genes that promote cell proliferation) and the inactivation of tumor suppressor genes (genes that inhibit cell growth and promote apoptosis). As cancer cells proliferate, they acquire additional mutations that enable them to evade immune surveillance, invade surrounding tissues, and metastasize to distant organs, leading to the spread of the disease.

The progression of cancer is a dynamic and heterogeneous process characterized by clonal evolution, genetic heterogeneity, and tumor microenvironment interactions. Cancer cells undergo selective pressure, adapting and evolving in response to changing environmental conditions, therapeutic interventions, and host immune responses. This complexity poses significant challenges for cancer diagnosis, treatment, and management.

Lifestyle Factors Influencing Cancer Development

While genetics plays a significant role in cancer susceptibility, accumulating evidence suggests that lifestyle factors play an equally important role in cancer development. Lifestyle choices, including diet, physical activity, tobacco use, alcohol consumption, stress management, and environmental exposures, can either promote or inhibit cancer initiation, progression, and recurrence.

1. **Diet:** A diet rich in fruits, vegetables, whole grains, lean proteins, and healthy fats is associated with a reduced risk of cancer, while a diet high in processed foods, red and processed meats, sugary beverages, and saturated fats is linked to an increased risk. Plant-based diets, in particular,

are rich in antioxidants, phytochemicals, and fiber, which have protective effects against cancer.

2. **Physical Activity:** Regular physical activity is associated with a lower risk of developing several types of cancer, including breast, colon, prostate, and lung cancer. Exercise helps maintain a healthy weight, reduces inflammation, improves immune function, and regulates hormone levels, all of which contribute to cancer prevention and control.

3. **Tobacco Use:** Tobacco use, including smoking and smokeless tobacco products, is the leading cause of preventable cancer deaths worldwide. Smoking is strongly linked to lung cancer, as well as cancers of the mouth, throat, esophagus, bladder, pancreas, and cervix. Quitting smoking significantly reduces the risk of developing cancer and improves overall health outcomes.

4. **Alcohol Consumption:** Heavy alcohol consumption is associated with an increased risk of several cancers, including those of the breast, liver, esophagus, throat, and mouth. Alcohol promotes carcinogenesis through various mechanisms, including the production of acetaldehyde (a toxic byproduct of alcohol metabolism), oxidative stress, and disruption of DNA repair mechanisms.

5. **Stress Management:** Chronic stress and psychological factors such as anxiety, depression, and social isolation are

associated with an increased risk of cancer and poorer outcomes in cancer patients. Stress management techniques such as meditation, mindfulness, yoga, and social support can help reduce stress levels and improve overall well-being.

6. **Environmental Exposures:** Environmental factors such as exposure to carcinogens, pollutants, radiation, and electromagnetic fields can increase the risk of cancer. Occupational exposures, air and water pollution, pesticides, heavy metals, and radiation from medical imaging or nuclear sources are examples of environmental factors that may contribute to cancer development.

Conclusion

Cancer is a complex and multifactorial disease influenced by a combination of genetic, environmental, and lifestyle factors. Understanding the disease process of cancer and the role of lifestyle factors in its development is essential for cancer prevention, early detection, and effective management. By adopting healthy lifestyle habits, including a balanced diet, regular physical activity, tobacco cessation, moderate alcohol consumption, stress management, and minimizing exposure to environmental toxins, individuals can reduce their risk of cancer and improve their overall health and well-being. Through education, awareness, and empowerment, we can work together to reduce the burden of cancer and promote a healthier future for all.

CHAPTER FIVE

The Power of Greens: Exploring the Nutritional Benefits of Leafy Greens and Herbs in Cancer Prevention and Treatment

Leafy greens and herbs are nutritional powerhouses that offer a wealth of health benefits, including cancer prevention and treatment support. Packed with vitamins, minerals, antioxidants, and phytochemicals, these vibrant green plants possess potent anti-inflammatory, immune-enhancing, and detoxifying properties that can play a significant role in reducing cancer risk and improving outcomes for those undergoing treatment. In this exploration, we delve into the nutritional benefits of leafy greens and herbs and their potential impact on cancer prevention and treatment.

Nutritional Benefits of Leafy Greens and Herbs

Leafy greens, such as spinach, kale, Swiss chard, collard greens, and arugula, are among the most nutrient-dense foods available, providing an abundance of vitamins, minerals, fiber, and phytonutrients essential for optimal health. Similarly, herbs such as parsley, cilantro, basil, mint, and dill are rich in vitamins, minerals, antioxidants, and essential oils that contribute to their medicinal properties.

1. **Vitamins and Minerals:** Leafy greens and herbs are excellent sources of vitamins A, C, K, and folate, as well as minerals like calcium, magnesium, potassium, and iron. These nutrients play crucial roles in immune function, antioxidant defense, bone health, blood clotting, and energy metabolism.

2. **Antioxidants:** Leafy greens and herbs are rich in antioxidants, including vitamins C and E, beta-carotene, lutein, zeaxanthin, and flavonoids. These compounds help neutralize harmful free radicals, reduce oxidative stress, and protect cells from DNA damage, inflammation, and chronic disease, including cancer.

3. **Phytochemicals:** Phytochemicals are bioactive compounds found in plants that have protective effects against cancer and other chronic diseases. Leafy greens and herbs contain a diverse array of phytochemicals, including glucosinolates, carotenoids, polyphenols, and flavonoids, which exert anti-inflammatory, antioxidant, anti-carcinogenic, and immune-enhancing effects.

4. **Fiber:** Leafy greens and herbs are rich in dietary fiber, which promotes digestive health, regulates blood sugar levels, supports weight management, and reduces the risk of colorectal cancer. Fiber also helps remove toxins and waste

products from the body, supporting detoxification and elimination processes.

Cancer Prevention and Treatment Support

The nutritional benefits of leafy greens and herbs make them valuable allies in cancer prevention and treatment support:

1. **Anti-Cancer Properties:** The phytochemicals found in leafy greens and herbs have been shown to possess anti-cancer properties by inhibiting tumor growth, inducing apoptosis (programmed cell death), preventing angiogenesis (the formation of new blood vessels to supply tumors), and reducing inflammation and oxidative stress.

2. **Immune Enhancement:** Leafy greens and herbs support immune function by providing essential nutrients and phytochemicals that strengthen the body's natural defense mechanisms against cancer cells and pathogens. A strong immune system is essential for detecting and eliminating abnormal cells before they develop into cancerous tumors.

3. **Detoxification Support:** Leafy greens and herbs contain compounds that support liver function and enhance detoxification processes, helping to eliminate carcinogens, toxins, and metabolic waste products from the body. Supporting the body's natural detoxification pathways is crucial for reducing cancer risk and promoting overall health.

4. **Anti-Inflammatory Effects:** Chronic inflammation plays a central role in cancer development and progression. Leafy greens and herbs possess anti-inflammatory properties that help reduce inflammation, inhibit the production of pro-inflammatory cytokines, and modulate immune responses, thereby reducing the risk of cancer and improving treatment outcomes.

Incorporating Leafy Greens and Herbs into the Diet

Incorporating leafy greens and herbs into the diet is easy and delicious:

1. **Salads:** Add leafy greens such as spinach, kale, arugula, and mixed greens to salads, along with fresh herbs like parsley, cilantro, basil, and mint, for a nutrient-packed meal.

2. **Smoothies:** Blend leafy greens like spinach or kale into smoothies with fruits, nuts, seeds, and herbs for a refreshing and nutritious beverage.

3. **Soups and Stews:** Add leafy greens such as Swiss chard, collard greens, or cabbage to soups, stews, and stir-fries for an extra dose of vitamins, minerals, and fiber.

4. **Herbal Teas:** Brew fresh herbs such as mint, basil, lemon balm, or chamomile into herbal teas for a soothing and health-promoting beverage.

5. **Garnishes:** Use fresh herbs as garnishes for soups, salads, entrees, and side dishes to add flavor, aroma, and nutritional value to your meals.

Conclusion

Leafy greens and herbs are nutritional powerhouses that offer a myriad of health benefits, including cancer prevention and treatment support. Rich in vitamins, minerals, antioxidants, and phytochemicals, these vibrant green plants possess potent anti-inflammatory, immune-enhancing, and detoxifying properties that can help reduce cancer risk, support immune function, and improve treatment outcomes. By incorporating leafy greens and herbs into your diet on a regular basis, you can nourish your body, promote optimal health, and reduce your risk of cancer and other chronic diseases.

CHAPTER SIX

Creating Healing Smoothie Recipes: Step-by-Step Instructions for Blending Nutrient-Dense Green Smoothies

Green smoothies are a delicious and convenient way to incorporate nutrient-dense ingredients into your diet, providing a wealth of vitamins, minerals, antioxidants, and phytochemicals to support overall health and well-being. With a few simple steps and some creative combinations, you can create healing smoothie recipes that nourish your body, boost your immune system, and promote vitality. Here's a step-by-step guide to blending nutrient-dense green smoothies:

Step 1: Choose Your Leafy Greens

Start by selecting a variety of leafy greens to serve as the base of your smoothie. Some popular options include spinach, kale, Swiss chard, collard greens, arugula, and romaine lettuce. Leafy greens are rich in vitamins, minerals, fiber, and antioxidants, making them essential for promoting optimal health and vitality.

Step 2: Add Fruits for Natural Sweetness

Next, add a variety of fruits to your smoothie to provide natural sweetness and flavor. Choose from options such as bananas, berries (strawberries, blueberries, raspberries, blackberries), mangoes, pineapples, apples, pears, or oranges. Fruits not only add sweetness to your smoothie but also contribute essential vitamins, minerals, fiber, and antioxidants.

Step 3: Incorporate Healthy Fats and Proteins

To make your smoothie more satisfying and nutritious, incorporate healthy fats and proteins into the mix. Options include avocados, nut butters (almond butter, peanut butter), seeds (chia seeds, flaxseeds, hemp seeds), nuts (walnuts, almonds), yogurt (Greek yogurt, coconut yogurt), or protein powder (plant-based or whey protein). Healthy fats and proteins help stabilize blood sugar levels, promote satiety, and provide sustained energy throughout the day.

Step 4: Boost with Superfoods and Nutrient-Rich Add-Ins

To supercharge your smoothie with extra nutrients and health benefits, consider adding superfoods and nutrient-rich add-ins. Options include spirulina, chlorella, wheatgrass powder, moringa powder, matcha powder, maca powder, cacao powder, bee pollen, turmeric, ginger, cinnamon, or acai berries. These superfoods are packed with antioxidants, phytochemicals, and essential nutrients that support immune function, reduce inflammation, and promote overall well-being.

Step 5: Choose a Liquid Base

Finally, choose a liquid base to blend your smoothie to the desired consistency. Options include water, coconut water, almond milk, coconut milk, oat milk, soy milk, or hemp milk. Feel free to adjust the amount of liquid based on your preference for a thicker or thinner smoothie consistency.

Step 6: Blend Until Smooth

Once you've added all your ingredients to the blender, secure the lid tightly and blend until smooth and creamy. Start at a low speed and gradually increase to high speed to ensure thorough blending. Pause occasionally to scrape down the sides of the blender and ensure all ingredients are incorporated evenly.

Step 7: Taste and Adjust

After blending, taste your smoothie and adjust the flavor and consistency as needed. You can add more fruits for sweetness, additional liquid for a thinner consistency, or extra superfoods for a nutritional boost. Get creative and experiment with different flavor combinations until you find your perfect healing smoothie recipe.

Step 8: Serve and Enjoy

Pour your freshly blended green smoothie into a glass or bowl and garnish with toppings such as fresh fruit slices, nuts, seeds, coconut flakes, or a drizzle of honey or maple syrup. Enjoy your healing smoothie as a nutritious breakfast, snack, or meal replacement, and feel the nourishing benefits as you sip and savor each delicious sip.

Conclusion

Creating healing smoothie recipes is a simple and enjoyable way to incorporate nutrient-dense ingredients into your diet and promote optimal health and vitality. By following these step-by-step instructions and getting creative with your combinations, you can blend delicious green smoothies that nourish your body, boost your immune system, and support your overall well-being. Cheers to your health and wellness journey!

CHAPTER SEVEN

Herbal Support for Cancer: Identifying Key Herbs and Supplements Recommended by Dr. Barbara for Cancer Care

Dr. Barbara, a respected figure in integrative medicine and holistic health, advocates for the use of herbs and supplements as part of a comprehensive approach to cancer care. Drawing on her extensive knowledge of herbal medicine and natural healing modalities, Dr. Barbara recommends a variety of herbs and supplements that have been shown to support the body's healing processes, enhance treatment outcomes, and improve quality of life for individuals living with cancer. In this guide, we'll explore some key herbs and supplements recommended by Dr. Barbara for cancer support:

1. Turmeric (Curcuma longa): Turmeric is a potent anti-inflammatory and antioxidant herb that has been extensively studied for its potential anti-cancer effects. Curcumin, the active compound in turmeric, has been shown to inhibit cancer cell growth, induce apoptosis (programmed cell death), and suppress tumor formation and metastasis. Dr. Barbara often recommends turmeric supplementation or incorporating fresh turmeric root into the diet to support cancer treatment and reduce inflammation.

2. Green Tea (Camellia sinensis): Green tea is rich in polyphenols, particularly epigallocatechin gallate (EGCG), which have been shown to possess anti-cancer properties. Green tea extract has been studied for its ability to inhibit tumor growth, angiogenesis (the formation of new blood vessels to supply tumors), and metastasis, as well as induce apoptosis in cancer cells. Dr. Barbara may recommend green tea supplementation or regular consumption of green tea as part of a cancer prevention and treatment regimen.

3. Medicinal Mushrooms: Certain mushrooms, such as reishi (Ganoderma lucidum), shiitake (Lentinula edodes), maitake (Grifolafrondosa), and turkey tail (Trametes versicolor), have been used for centuries in traditional medicine for their immune-modulating and anti-cancer properties. These mushrooms contain bioactive compounds such as beta-glucans, polysaccharides, and triterpenes that support immune function, enhance chemotherapy and radiation therapy efficacy, and improve quality of life for cancer patients. Dr. Barbara may recommend mushroom supplements or incorporating medicinal mushrooms into the diet to support cancer treatment.

4. Astragalus (Astragalus membranaceus): Astragalus is an adaptogenic herb that has been used in traditional Chinese medicine for centuries to strengthen the immune system, improve energy levels, and enhance overall vitality. Astragalus contains polysaccharides and flavonoids that stimulate the production of white blood cells, enhance immune function, and increase resistance to infections and disease. Dr. Barbara may recommend astragalus supplementation or incorporating astragalus root into herbal formulas to support immune function during cancer treatment.

5. Milk Thistle (Silybum marianum): Milk thistle is a well-known herb with hepatoprotective properties, traditionally used to support liver health and detoxification. Silymarin, the active compound in milk thistle, has antioxidant and anti-inflammatory effects and may help protect the liver from damage caused by cancer treatments such as chemotherapy and radiation therapy. Dr. Barbara may recommend milk thistle supplementation to support liver function and reduce treatment-related side effects in cancer patients.

6. Essiac Tea: Essiac tea is a traditional herbal remedy consisting of a blend of herbs, including burdock root, sheep sorrel, slippery elm bark, and Indian rhubarb root, that has been used for decades as an alternative cancer treatment. While scientific evidence supporting the efficacy of Essiac tea for cancer is limited, some studies suggest that it may have immune-modulating, antioxidant, and anti-inflammatory effects that could potentially benefit cancer patients. Dr. Barbara may recommend

Essiac tea as an adjunctive therapy for individuals seeking complementary approaches to cancer treatment.

7. Vitamin D: Vitamin D plays a crucial role in immune function, inflammation regulation, and cellular growth and differentiation, making it an important nutrient for cancer prevention and treatment. Low levels of vitamin D have been associated with an increased risk of certain cancers and poorer outcomes in cancer patients. Dr. Barbara may recommend vitamin D supplementation or regular sun exposure to maintain optimal vitamin D levels and support overall health and well-being in individuals living with cancer.

8. Omega-3 Fatty Acids: Omega-3 fatty acids, found in fatty fish (such as salmon, mackerel, and sardines), flaxseeds, chia seeds, and walnuts, have anti-inflammatory and anti-cancer properties that may benefit individuals with cancer. Omega-3 fatty acids have been shown to inhibit tumor growth, reduce inflammation, and enhance the effectiveness of chemotherapy and radiation therapy. Dr. Barbara may recommend omega-3 supplements or incorporating omega-3-rich foods into the diet to support cancer treatment and improve quality of life.

Important Considerations:

- Before starting any herbal supplements or complementary therapies, it's essential to consult with a qualified healthcare practitioner, such as an integrative oncologist, naturopathic doctor, or herbalist, who can provide personalized recommendations based on your individual health status, cancer diagnosis, treatment plan, and goals.

- Herbal supplements can interact with medications and treatments, so it's important to inform your healthcare provider of all supplements you are taking to avoid potential adverse effects or interactions.

- While herbs and supplements can play a valuable role in supporting cancer treatment and improving quality of life, they should not be used as a substitute for conventional medical care. It's essential to integrate complementary therapies into a comprehensive cancer care plan that includes conventional treatments such as surgery, chemotherapy, radiation therapy, and supportive care.

- It's also important to maintain a healthy lifestyle, including a balanced diet, regular exercise, stress management, adequate sleep, and avoidance of tobacco and excessive alcohol consumption, to optimize cancer treatment outcomes and promote overall well-being.

In conclusion, herbal support can be a valuable adjunctive therapy for individuals undergoing cancer treatment, offering immune-enhancing, anti-inflammatory, antioxidant, and supportive effects that complement conventional medical care. By working with a qualified healthcare provider and incorporating herbs and supplements into a comprehensive cancer care plan, individuals can support their body's healing processes, improve treatment outcomes, and enhance their overall quality of life.

CHAPTER EIGHT

Integrating Smoothies into Cancer Treatment Plans: Practical Strategies for Incorporating Smoothies into a Healing Diet

Smoothies offer a convenient and nutritious way to incorporate essential nutrients into the diet, making them an excellent option for individuals undergoing cancer treatment. Whether as a meal replacement, snack, or supplement, smoothies can provide much-needed hydration, nourishment, and support during cancer therapy. In this guide, we'll explore practical strategies for integrating smoothies into cancer treatment plans and optimizing their nutritional benefits for healing and recovery.

1. Tailor Recipes to Individual Preferences and Needs:

When incorporating smoothies into a cancer treatment plan, it's essential to tailor recipes to individual preferences, dietary restrictions, and treatment-related side effects. Consider factors such as taste preferences, texture preferences (e.g., thick vs. thin), food intolerances or allergies, appetite changes, nausea, difficulty swallowing, and mouth sores. For example, individuals experiencing nausea may prefer lighter, fruit-based smoothies with ginger or mint to help alleviate symptoms, while those with appetite loss may benefit from denser, protein-rich smoothies with nut butters or protein powder to increase caloric intake.

2. Focus on Nutrient-Dense Ingredients:

Choose nutrient-dense ingredients for your smoothies to maximize their nutritional benefits. Include a variety of fruits, vegetables, leafy greens, herbs, healthy fats, proteins, and superfoods to provide a broad spectrum of vitamins, minerals, antioxidants, phytochemicals, fiber, and essential nutrients. Aim to include a balance of macronutrients (carbohydrates, proteins, fats) and micronutrients (vitamins, minerals) to support overall health and well-being during cancer treatment.

3. Experiment with Flavor Combinations and Add-Ins:

Get creative with your smoothie recipes by experimenting with different flavor combinations and add-ins to suit individual tastes and nutritional needs. Consider incorporating herbs, spices, extracts, and flavorings such as cinnamon, vanilla, mint, ginger, turmeric, and citrus zest to enhance flavor and aroma. Explore a variety of fruits, vegetables, leafy greens, and superfoods such as berries, bananas, avocados, spinach, kale, chia seeds, flaxseeds, hemp seeds, and coconut flakes to add nutritional diversity and complexity to your smoothies.

4. Customize Texture and Consistency:

Adjust the texture and consistency of your smoothies to accommodate individual preferences and needs. Experiment with different ratios of liquid to solid ingredients to achieve your desired thickness and smoothness. For individuals experiencing difficulty swallowing or mouth sores, consider blending smoothies to a thinner consistency or straining them to remove fibrous pulp. Alternatively, adding creamy ingredients such as yogurt, nut butters, avocado, or coconut milk can help create a smoother texture and enhance palatability.

5. Incorporate Functional Ingredients for Specific Needs:

Include functional ingredients in your smoothies to address specific nutritional needs or treatment-related side effects. For example, adding protein powder or Greek yogurt can help support muscle strength and repair during cancer treatment. Including omega-3-rich foods such as chia seeds, flaxseeds, or walnuts can help reduce inflammation and support cognitive function. Adding fiber-rich ingredients such as oats, psyllium husk, or ground flaxseeds can promote digestive health and regularity. Consider incorporating adaptogenic herbs such as ashwagandha, holy basil, or rhodiola to help reduce stress and support overall resilience during cancer therapy.

6. Schedule Regular Smoothie Times for Consistency:

Establish a routine for incorporating smoothies into your daily schedule to ensure consistency and adherence. Schedule regular smoothie times throughout the day, such as breakfast, mid-morning snack, lunch, or afternoon snack, to provide consistent nourishment and support energy levels. Prepare smoothies in advance and store them in individual portions in the refrigerator or freezer for quick and convenient access, especially during times when appetite may be low or energy levels are depleted.

7. Hydrate and Stay Well-Nourished:

Incorporate hydrating ingredients into your smoothies to help maintain optimal hydration levels during cancer treatment. Include water, coconut water, herbal teas, or hydrating fruits and vegetables such as cucumbers, celery, melons, and citrus fruits to ensure adequate fluid intake. Additionally, focus on incorporating nutrient-rich ingredients into your smoothies to support overall nourishment, energy levels, and well-being. Aim to include a balance of carbohydrates, proteins, and healthy fats to provide sustained energy and support muscle strength and repair.

8. Monitor Symptoms and Adjust Recipes Accordingly:

Pay attention to how your body responds to different smoothie recipes and ingredients, and adjust your recipes accordingly based on your symptoms and preferences. If certain ingredients exacerbate nausea, digestive discomfort, or other side effects, consider removing or substituting them with more tolerable alternatives. Similarly, if you find certain flavor combinations or textures more appealing, prioritize those in your smoothie recipes to enhance palatability and enjoyment.

In conclusion, integrating smoothies into cancer treatment plans can provide valuable support and nourishment during therapy. By tailoring recipes to individual preferences and needs, focusing on nutrient-dense ingredients, experimenting with flavor combinations and textures, incorporating functional ingredients, scheduling regular smoothie times, staying hydrated, and monitoring symptoms, individuals can optimize the nutritional benefits of smoothies and enhance their overall quality of life during cancer treatment.

CHAPTER NINE

Testimonials of Healing: Inspiring Stories of Individuals Who Have Experienced Cancer Remission with Dr. Barbara's Smoothies

Dr. Barbara's holistic approach to cancer care, including the incorporation of nutrient-dense smoothies into treatment plans, has yielded remarkable results for many individuals facing cancer diagnosis and treatment. These inspiring testimonials highlight the transformative power of Dr. Barbara's smoothies in supporting cancer remission and improving quality of life for patients on their healing journeys.

1. Sarah's Story: Overcoming Breast Cancer

Sarah, a 45-year-old mother of two, was diagnosed with stage II breast cancer and underwent surgery, chemotherapy, and radiation therapy as part of her treatment plan. Despite conventional treatments, Sarah experienced debilitating side effects such as fatigue, nausea, and loss of appetite, making it challenging to maintain adequate nutrition and energy levels.

Desperate for relief, Sarah turned to Dr. Barbara's holistic approach to cancer care, which included incorporating nutrient-dense smoothies into her daily routine. With Dr. Barbara's guidance, Sarah began blending a variety of fruits, vegetables, leafy greens, and superfoods into delicious and nourishing smoothies that provided essential nutrients and hydration to support her body's healing processes.

Over time, Sarah noticed a significant improvement in her energy levels, appetite, and overall well-being. The nutrient-rich smoothies helped alleviate her treatment-related side effects, boost her immune system, and enhance her resilience during chemotherapy and radiation therapy. With the support of Dr. Barbara's smoothies and holistic therapies, Sarah successfully completed her cancer treatment and achieved remission, inspiring hope and resilience in others facing similar challenges.

2. Mark's Journey: Thriving After Prostate Cancer

Mark, a 60-year-old retiree, was diagnosed with localized prostate cancer and opted for surgery followed by radiation therapy as his primary treatment approach. While the treatments were successful in removing the cancerous tumor and preventing its recurrence, Mark experienced lingering side effects such as urinary incontinence, erectile dysfunction, and fatigue that affected his quality of life.

Seeking additional support for his recovery, Mark turned to Dr. Barbara's integrative approach to cancer care, which emphasized the importance of nutrition, lifestyle modifications, and complementary therapies in promoting healing and well-being. Inspired by Dr. Barbara's recommendations, Mark began incorporating nutrient-dense smoothies into his daily routine as a way to nourish his body, support his immune system, and optimize his recovery.

With Dr. Barbara's guidance, Mark experimented with different smoothie recipes tailored to his nutritional needs and preferences, incorporating ingredients such as berries, leafy greens, flaxseeds, Greek yogurt, and turmeric to enhance his overall health and vitality. Over time, Mark noticed a remarkable improvement in his energy levels, urinary function, and overall quality of life, thanks to the healing power of Dr. Barbara's smoothies and holistic approach to cancer recovery.

Today, Mark continues to thrive post-cancer treatment, enjoying an active and fulfilling life thanks to the transformative impact of Dr. Barbara's smoothies and integrative therapies on his journey to wellness.

3. Emily's Triumph: Beating Leukemia Against All Odds

Emily, a 12-year-old girl, was diagnosed with acute lymphoblastic leukemia (ALL), a rare and aggressive form of childhood cancer. Despite undergoing intensive chemotherapy and bone marrow transplant, Emily's prognosis remained uncertain, and her family was devastated by the challenges and uncertainties of her cancer journey.

Determined to support Emily's healing and recovery, her parents sought out alternative therapies and nutritional interventions to complement her conventional cancer treatment. They discovered Dr. Barbara's holistic approach to cancer care, which emphasized the importance of nutrition, immune support, and holistic healing modalities in promoting cancer remission and overall well-being.

With Dr. Barbara's guidance, Emily's parents began incorporating nutrient-dense smoothies into her daily diet, packed with immune-boosting ingredients such as berries, spinach, avocado, and medicinal mushrooms. The smoothies provided essential nutrients, hydration, and support for Emily's immune system, helping her body withstand the rigors of chemotherapy and recover from the effects of treatment.

Despite the odds, Emily responded positively to the integrative approach to cancer care, experiencing fewer treatment-related side effects, faster recovery times, and improved overall health and vitality. With the support of Dr. Barbara's smoothies and holistic therapies, Emily successfully completed her cancer treatment and achieved remission, inspiring hope and resilience in others facing similar challenges.

These testimonials are just a few examples of the countless individuals who have experienced cancer remission and improved quality of life with the support of Dr. Barbara's smoothies and holistic approach to cancer care. Through personalized guidance, nutritional support, and compassionate care, Dr. Barbara continues to empower patients on their healing journeys and inspire hope for a brighter, healthier future beyond cancer.

CHAPTER TEN

Beyond Cancer: Sustaining Overall Health and Wellness Through Long-Term Preventive Practices and Dietary Habits

While cancer treatment focuses on addressing the immediate challenges of diagnosis and recovery, sustaining overall health and wellness in the long term requires a proactive approach to preventive practices and dietary habits. By adopting lifestyle changes and nutritional strategies that promote health and vitality, individuals can reduce their risk of cancer recurrence, enhance their quality of life, and support their long-term well-being. In this guide, we'll explore key preventive practices and dietary habits to help individuals sustain overall health and wellness beyond cancer.

1. Maintain a Balanced Diet:

A balanced diet rich in fruits, vegetables, whole grains, lean proteins, and healthy fats forms the foundation of long-term health and wellness. Aim to include a variety of colorful fruits and vegetables in your daily meals to provide essential vitamins, minerals, antioxidants, and phytonutrients that support immune function, reduce inflammation, and protect against cancer and other chronic diseases. Choose whole grains such as brown rice, quinoa, oats, and whole wheat bread over refined grains to increase fiber intake and promote digestive health. Incorporate lean proteins such as poultry, fish, beans, lentils, and tofu to support muscle strength and repair. Include healthy fats from sources such as avocados, nuts, seeds, and olive oil to support heart health, brain function, and overall well-being.

2. Stay Active and Exercise Regularly:

Regular physical activity is essential for maintaining overall health and reducing the risk of cancer recurrence and other chronic diseases. Aim for at least 150 minutes of moderate-intensity aerobic exercise or 75 minutes of vigorous-intensity aerobic exercise per week, along with muscle-strengthening activities on two or more days per week. Incorporate a variety of activities such as walking, jogging, cycling, swimming, yoga, and strength training to improve cardiovascular health, muscle tone, flexibility, and balance. Find activities that you enjoy and make them a regular part of your routine to promote long-term adherence and sustainability.

3. Manage Stress and Prioritize Self-Care:

Chronic stress can negatively impact immune function, inflammation levels, and overall health, increasing the risk of cancer recurrence and other health problems. Prioritize self-care practices such as mindfulness meditation, deep breathing exercises, yoga, tai chi, journaling, and relaxation techniques to reduce stress levels and promote emotional well-being. Make time for activities that bring you joy and relaxation, such as spending time in nature, engaging in hobbies, connecting with loved ones, and pursuing creative outlets. Set boundaries, delegate tasks, and practice saying no to avoid overcommitment and overwhelm, allowing yourself time to recharge and rejuvenate.

4. Avoid Tobacco and Limit Alcohol Consumption:

Tobacco use is the leading cause of preventable cancer deaths worldwide, increasing the risk of several types of cancer, including lung, mouth, throat, esophagus, bladder, pancreas, and cervix. If you smoke or use tobacco products, seek support and resources to quit smoking and reduce your risk of cancer and other health problems. Additionally, limit alcohol consumption to moderate levels, defined as up to one drink per day for women and up to two drinks per day for men, to reduce the risk of cancer, liver disease, and other health complications associated with excessive alcohol intake.

5. Practice Sun Safety and Skin Protection:

Excessive sun exposure and ultraviolet (UV) radiation can increase the risk of skin cancer, including melanoma, basal cell carcinoma, and squamous cell carcinoma. Protect your skin from the sun's harmful rays by wearing sunscreen with a sun protection factor (SPF) of 30 or higher, seeking shade during peak sun hours, wearing protective clothing such as hats and sunglasses, and avoiding indoor tanning beds and sunlamps. Perform regular skin self-exams to monitor for changes in moles, freckles, or other skin lesions and seek prompt medical attention for any concerning symptoms or abnormalities.

6. Stay Connected and Cultivate Supportive Relationships:

Social support and connectedness are essential for maintaining overall health and wellness, especially during times of illness or recovery. Stay connected with friends, family, and loved ones through regular communication, social activities, and meaningful interactions. Join support groups, online communities, or local organizations to connect with others who share similar experiences and provide mutual encouragement, understanding, and support. Cultivate relationships that uplift and inspire you, surround yourself with positive influences, and seek help when needed to navigate challenges and overcome obstacles on your journey to long-term health and well-being.

Conclusion:

Sustaining overall health and wellness beyond cancer requires a multifaceted approach that encompasses preventive practices, dietary habits, and lifestyle changes aimed at promoting long-term vitality and resilience. By maintaining a balanced diet, staying active and exercising regularly, managing stress and prioritizing self-care, avoiding tobacco and limiting alcohol consumption, practicing sun safety and skin protection, and staying connected and cultivating supportive relationships, individuals can reduce their risk of cancer recurrence, enhance their quality of life, and enjoy lasting health and well-being for years to come. Through proactive self-care and mindful living, individuals can empower themselves to live fully and thrive beyond cancer, embracing each day with gratitude, resilience, and hope for a brighter future.

CHAPTEER 11

DR. BARBARA GREEN SMOOTHIES FOR CANCER CURE

1. Spinach and Kale Detox Smoothie

Definition: A nutrient-packed smoothie designed to detoxify the body and boost immune function.

Ingredients: 1 cup spinach, 1 cup kale, 1 banana, 1 cup almond milk, 1 tbsp chia seeds, 1 tbsp honey.

How to Prepare: Blend all ingredients until smooth.

How it Works: Spinach and kale are rich in antioxidants and phytonutrients that may help protect cells from damage.

How to Use: Drink once daily, preferably in the morning.

Dosage: 1 large glass (about 12 oz).

Side Effects: May cause mild digestive discomfort if not used to high fiber intake.

Precautions: Ensure greens are washed thoroughly to avoid contamination.

2. Broccoli and Apple Smoothie

Definition: A green smoothie focusing on the cancer-fighting properties of broccoli.

Ingredients: 1 cup broccoli florets, 1 apple, 1 cup spinach, 1/2 lemon (juiced), 1 cup water.

How to Prepare: Blend all ingredients until smooth.

How it Works: Broccoli contains sulforaphane, a compound with potential anticancer properties.

How to Use: Consume once daily.

Dosage: 1 large glass.

Side Effects: May cause gas or bloating.

Precautions: Introduce broccoli gradually if sensitive to cruciferous vegetables.

3. Cucumber and Mint Smoothie

Definition: A refreshing smoothie to hydrate and provide antioxidants. **Ingredients:** 1 cucumber, 1 cup spinach, a handful of mint leaves, 1/2 lime (juiced), 1 cup coconut water.

How to Prepare: Blend until smooth.

How it Works: Cucumbers are hydrating and provide flavonoids; mint aids digestion.

How to Use: Drink in the afternoon or after meals.

Dosage: 1 large glass. **Side Effects:** Generally well-tolerated.

Precautions: Monitor for any allergic reactions to mint.

4. Celery and Ginger Smoothie

Definition: A smoothie to support detoxification and digestion. **Ingredients:** 2 stalks celery, 1/2 inch ginger, 1 cup spinach, 1 green apple, 1 cup water.

How to Prepare: Blend until smooth. **How it Works:** Ginger has anti-inflammatory and anticancer properties.

How to Use: Consume in the morning.

 Dosage: 1 large glass.

Side Effects: May cause mild digestive discomfort.

Precautions: Avoid ginger if on blood thinners.

5. Avocado and Kale Smoothie

Definition: A creamy smoothie rich in healthy fats and nutrients. **Ingredients:** 1/2 avocado, 1 cup kale, 1 banana, 1 cup unsweetened almond milk, 1 tbsp flaxseeds.

How to Prepare: Blend until smooth.

How it Works: Avocado provides healthy fats and antioxidants.

How to Use: Drink as a meal replacement.

Dosage: 1 large glass.

Side Effects: Generally well-tolerated.

Precautions: Watch for calorie intake if weight management is a concern.

6. Green Apple and Spinach Smoothie

Definition: A smoothie to boost immunity and provide fiber.
Ingredients: 1 green apple, 1 cup spinach, 1/2 cucumber, 1 tbsp lemon juice, 1 cup water.

How to Prepare: Blend until smooth.

How it Works: Apples provide pectin, which may support gut health.

How to Use: Drink mid-morning or mid-afternoon.

Dosage: 1 large glass.

Side Effects: May cause gas or bloating.

Precautions: Introduce high-fiber ingredients gradually.

7. Parsley and Pineapple Smoothie

Definition: A detoxifying and anti-inflammatory smoothie.
Ingredients: A handful of parsley, 1 cup pineapple chunks, 1 cup spinach, 1/2 banana, 1 cup coconut water.

How to Prepare: Blend until smooth.

How it Works: Parsley is rich in vitamins and has diuretic properties.

How to Use: Consume in the morning.

Dosage: 1 large glass.

Side Effects: Parsley may act as a diuretic.

Precautions: Avoid excessive parsley if pregnant or on blood thinners.

8. Green Tea and Mango Smoothie

Definition: An antioxidant-rich smoothie to enhance overall health.

Ingredients: 1 cup brewed green tea (cooled), 1 cup mango chunks, 1 cup spinach, 1 tbsp chia seeds.

How to Prepare: Blend until smooth.

How it Works: Green tea contains catechins with potential anticancer properties.

How to Use: Drink in the morning.

Dosage: 1 large glass.

Side Effects: May cause mild caffeine-related side effects.

Precautions: Avoid before bedtime due to caffeine content.

9. Spirulina and Banana Smoothie

Definition: A nutrient-dense smoothie with added protein and minerals.

Ingredients: 1 tsp spirulina powder, 1 banana, 1 cup spinach, 1 cup almond milk, 1 tbsp honey.

How to Prepare: Blend until smooth.

How it Works: Spirulina is a potent source of antioxidants and protein.

How to Use: Drink as a meal replacement.

Dosage: 1 large glass.

Side Effects: May cause mild digestive discomfort initially.

Precautions: Start with small amounts of spirulina.

10. Wheatgrass and Kiwi Smoothie

Definition: A detoxifying smoothie with high chlorophyll content.
Ingredients: 1 tbsp wheatgrass juice or powder, 2 kiwis, 1 cup spinach, 1 cup coconut water.

How to Prepare: Blend until smooth.

How it Works: Wheatgrass is known for its detoxifying and antioxidant properties.

 How to Use: Drink in the morning.

Dosage: 1 large glass.

Side Effects: May cause nausea if taken in excess.

Precautions: Start with small amounts of wheatgrass.

11. Carrot and Kale Smoothie

Definition: A beta-carotene-rich smoothie for immune support.
Ingredients: 2 carrots, 1 cup kale, 1 orange, 1 cup water, 1 tbsp flaxseed oil.

How to Prepare: Blend until smooth.

How it Works: Carrots provide beta-carotene, which supports immune function.

How to Use: Consume in the morning.

Dosage: 1 large glass.

Side Effects: Generally well-tolerated.

Precautions: Consume in moderation to avoid excessive vitamin A intake.

12. Beet and Spinach Smoothie

Definition: A detoxifying and blood-boosting smoothie. **Ingredients:** 1 small beet, 1 cup spinach, 1 apple, 1/2 lemon (juiced), 1 cup water.

How to Prepare: Blend until smooth.

How it Works: Beets support liver function and provide antioxidants.

How to Use: Drink mid-morning.

Dosage: 1 large glass.

Side Effects: May cause red urine or stool.

Precautions: Monitor for any allergic reactions to beets.

13. Aloe Vera and Green Apple Smoothie

Definition: A soothing smoothie for digestion and hydration.
Ingredients: 1 tbsp aloe vera gel, 1 green apple, 1 cup spinach, 1/2 cucumber, 1 cup water.

How to Prepare: Blend until smooth.

How it Works: Aloe vera supports digestive health and has anti-inflammatory properties.

How to Use: Drink in the afternoon. **Dosage:** 1 large glass.

Side Effects: May cause digestive discomfort if taken in excess.

Precautions: Ensure aloe vera is pure and safe for consumption.

14. Dandelion Greens and Pear Smoothie

Definition: A liver-supporting and detoxifying smoothie.
Ingredients: 1 cup dandelion greens, 1 pear, 1/2 lemon (juiced), 1 cup water.

How to Prepare: Blend until smooth.

How it Works: Dandelion greens support liver detoxification.

How to Use: Drink in the morning.

Dosage: 1 large glass.

Side Effects: May act as a diuretic.

Precautions: Avoid if allergic to dandelion.

15. Chlorella and Pineapple Smoothie

Definition: A detoxifying and nutrient-rich smoothie.

Ingredients: 1 tsp chlorella powder, 1 cup pineapple chunks, 1 cup spinach, 1 cup coconut water.

How to Prepare: Blend until smooth.

How it Works: Chlorella is known for its detoxifying properties.

How to Use: Drink in the morning.

Dosage: 1 large glass.

Side Effects: May cause mild digestive discomfort.

Precautions: Start with small amounts of chlorella.

16. Collard Greens and Peach Smoothie

Definition: A vitamin-rich smoothie for immune support.
Ingredients: 1 cup collard greens, 1 peach, 1 banana, 1 cup almond milk.

How to Prepare: Blend until smooth.

How it Works: Collard greens are high in vitamins A, C, and K.

How to Use: Drink mid-morning.

Dosage: 1 large glass.

Side Effects: Generally well-tolerated.

Precautions: Ensure thorough washing of collard greens.

17. Swiss Chard and Blueberry Smoothie

Definition: An antioxidant-rich smoothie for overall health.
Ingredients: 1 cup Swiss chard, 1 cup blueberries, 1 banana, 1 cup water.

How to Prepare: Blend until smooth.

How it Works: Blueberries provide powerful antioxidants.

How to Use: Drink in the afternoon. **Dosage:** 1 large glass.

Side Effects: Generally well-tolerated.

Precautions: Watch for any allergic reactions to berries.

18. Matcha and Banana Smoothie

Definition: A smoothie to boost energy and provide antioxidants.

Ingredients: 1 tsp matcha powder, 1 banana, 1 cup spinach, 1 cup almond milk.

How to Prepare: Blend until smooth.

How it Works: Matcha provides concentrated antioxidants and a mild caffeine boost.

How to Use: Drink in the morning.

Dosage: 1 large glass.

Side Effects: May cause mild caffeine-related side effects.

Precautions: Avoid before bedtime due to caffeine content.

19. Arugula and Melon Smoothie

Definition: A refreshing and hydrating smoothie.

Ingredients: 1 cup arugula, 1 cup melon (honeydew or cantaloupe), 1/2 lime (juiced), 1 cup water.

How to Prepare: Blend until smooth.

How it Works: Arugula provides vitamins and phytonutrients.

How to Use: Drink mid-morning.

Dosage: 1 large glass.

Side Effects: Generally well-tolerated.

Precautions: Ensure thorough washing of arugula.

20. Green Papaya and Spinach Smoothie

Definition: A digestive-supporting smoothie rich in enzymes. **Ingredients:** 1 cup green papaya, 1 cup spinach, 1 banana, 1 cup coconut water.

How to Prepare: Blend until smooth.

How it Works: Green papaya provides digestive enzymes.

How to Use: Drink before meals. **Dosage:** 1 large glass.

Side Effects: Generally well-tolerated.

Precautions: Avoid if allergic to papaya.

21. Zucchini and Apple Smoothie

Definition: A low-calorie smoothie for hydration and fiber. **Ingredients:** 1 small zucchini, 1 apple, 1 cup spinach, 1/2 lemon (juiced), 1 cup water.

How to Prepare: Blend until smooth.

How it Works: Zucchini is hydrating and provides fiber.

How to Use: Drink in the afternoon. **Dosage:** 1 large glass.

Side Effects: Generally well-tolerated.

Precautions: Ensure thorough washing of zucchini.

22. Bok Choy and Pineapple Smoothie

Definition: A nutrient-dense smoothie for immune support.

Ingredients: 1 cup bok choy, 1 cup pineapple chunks, 1/2 banana, 1 cup coconut water.

How to Prepare: Blend until smooth. **How it Works:** Bok choy is rich in vitamins A, C, and K.

How to Use: Drink mid-morning.

Dosage: 1 large glass.

Side Effects: Generally well-tolerated.

Precautions: Ensure thorough washing of bok choy.

23. Green Pepper and Mango Smoothie

Definition: A vitamin C-rich smoothie for immune support.

Ingredients: 1 green bell pepper, 1 cup mango chunks, 1 cup spinach, 1 cup water.

How to Prepare: Blend until smooth.

How it Works: Green bell peppers provide high levels of vitamin C.

How to Use: Drink in the morning. **Dosage:** 1 large glass.

Side Effects: May cause mild digestive discomfort.

Precautions: Ensure thorough washing of bell pepper.

24. Fennel and Apple Smoothie

Definition: A digestive-supporting and refreshing smoothie.

Ingredients: 1 small fennel bulb, 1 apple, 1 cup spinach, 1/2 lemon (juiced), 1 cup water.

How to Prepare: Blend until smooth.

How it Works: Fennel aids digestion and reduces inflammation.

How to Use: Drink before meals.

Dosage: 1 large glass. **Side Effects:** Generally well-tolerated.

Precautions: Avoid if allergic to fennel.

25. Turnip Greens and Strawberry Smoothie

Definition: A vitamin-rich smoothie for immune support.

Ingredients: 1 cup turnip greens, 1 cup strawberries, 1 banana, 1 cup almond milk. **How to Prepare:** Blend until smooth.

How it Works: Turnip greens provide vitamins A, C, and K.

How to Use: Drink mid-morning.

Dosage: 1 large glass. **Side Effects:** Generally well-tolerated.

Precautions: Ensure thorough washing of turnip greens.

BONUS: SOME HERBAL AND HOLISTIC REMEDIES TO KNOW

Bromide Plus Powder:

Definition: Bromide Plus Powder is a dietary supplement formulated to support thyroid health and promote overall well-being. It typically contains a blend of herbs and minerals that are believed to have beneficial effects on thyroid function.

Ingredients: Bromide Plus Powder often contains a combination of herbs such as bladderwrack, sea moss, and burdock root, along with minerals like iodine and potassium phosphate. These ingredients are thought to support thyroid function and maintain optimal iodine levels in the body.

How to Prepare: Bromide Plus Powder is usually mixed with water or juice to create a drinkable solution. It's important to follow the instructions on the product label for dosage and preparation.

Dosage: The dosage of Bromide Plus Powder can vary depending on the specific product and individual needs. It's crucial to consult with a healthcare professional or follow the recommended dosage on the product label to avoid potential side effects.

How to Use: Bromide Plus Powder is typically taken orally by mixing the recommended dosage with water or juice. It's important to shake or stir the mixture well before consuming it to ensure even distribution of the ingredients.

Side Effects: While Bromide Plus Powder is generally considered safe when used as directed, some individuals may experience side effects such as digestive discomfort or allergic reactions to certain ingredients. It's essential to consult with a healthcare provider before starting any new supplement regimen, especially if you have underlying health conditions or are taking medications.

Bugleweed:

Definition: Bugleweed, also known as Lycopusvirginicus, is a perennial herb native to North America and Europe. It has been used in traditional medicine to treat various conditions, including hyperthyroidism, anxiety, and insomnia.

Ingredients: Bugleweed contains several active compounds, including lithospermic acid, phenolic acids, and flavonoids. These compounds are believed to contribute to the herb's medicinal properties, particularly its ability to regulate thyroid function.

How to Prepare: Bugleweed is commonly consumed as a tea or tincture. To make tea, dried bugleweed leaves and flowers are steeped in hot water for several minutes before being strained and consumed. Tinctures are prepared by steeping the herb in alcohol or vinegar to extract its active compounds.

Dosage: The appropriate dosage of bugleweed can vary depending on factors such as age, health status, and the specific preparation being used. It's important to follow the recommended dosage on the product label or consult with a qualified herbalist or healthcare professional for personalized guidance.

How to Use: Bugleweed tea or tincture is typically taken orally. It can be consumed on its own or mixed with honey or other herbal teas for added flavor.

Side Effects: While bugleweed is generally considered safe for most people when used in moderation, excessive intake may cause digestive upset or allergic reactions in some individuals. Pregnant or breastfeeding women should avoid bugleweed due to its potential to stimulate uterine contractions. As with any herbal remedy, it's important to consult with a healthcare provider before using bugleweed, especially if you have underlying health conditions or are taking medications.

Burdock:

Definition: Burdock, scientifically known as Arctium lappa, is a biennial plant native to Europe and Asia but now found worldwide. It's part of the Asteraceae family and has been used for centuries in traditional medicine and culinary practices.

Ingredients: Burdock contains various nutrients, including carbohydrates, fiber, vitamins (such as vitamin B6, folate, and vitamin C), and minerals (including potassium, magnesium, and manganese). It also contains active compounds such as polyphenols and volatile oils.

How to Prepare: Burdock can be prepared and consumed in various ways. The roots, leaves, and seeds are all utilized for different purposes. The root is commonly used in cooking, herbal teas, tinctures, and supplements, while the leaves and seeds are sometimes used in herbal preparations.

Dosage: The appropriate dosage of burdock root can vary depending on the specific form and intended use. For culinary purposes, there are no strict dosage guidelines, but for supplements or herbal remedies, it's essential to follow the recommended dosage on the product label or consult with a healthcare professional.

How to Use: Burdock root can be used in cooking by peeling, slicing, and adding it to soups, stews, stir-fries, or salads. It can also be brewed into a tea or used to make tinctures or extracts for medicinal purposes. Some people may also take burdock root supplements in capsule or powder form.

Side Effects: While burdock is generally considered safe for most people when consumed in moderate amounts, some individuals may experience allergic reactions or digestive upset. Additionally, burdock may interact with certain medications or have adverse effects in individuals with certain health conditions, such as diabetes or allergies to plants in the Asteraceae family. It's important to consult with a healthcare provider before using burdock, especially if you have underlying health conditions or are taking medications.

Cascara Sagrada:

Definition: Cascara Sagrada, scientifically known as Rhamnus purshiana, is a species of buckthorn native to western North America. It has been used traditionally as a laxative and to promote bowel regularity.

Ingredients: The primary active ingredients in cascara sagrada are anthraquinone glycosides, particularly cascarosides A and B. These compounds stimulate peristalsis in the colon, leading to increased bowel movements.

How to Prepare: Cascara sagrada is typically prepared as an herbal tea, tincture, or capsule. To make tea, dried cascara sagrada bark is steeped in hot water for several minutes before being strained and consumed. Tinctures are prepared by steeping the bark in alcohol to extract its active compounds.

Dosage: The appropriate dosage of cascara sagrada can vary depending on the specific preparation and intended use. It's important to follow the recommended dosage on the product label or consult with a healthcare professional for personalized guidance.

How to Use: Cascara sagrada tea or tincture is typically taken orally. It's important to start with a low dose and gradually increase if needed to avoid potential side effects such as cramping or diarrhea.

Side Effects: Cascara sagrada is considered safe for short-term use when used as directed. However, long-term or excessive use may lead to dependence, electrolyte imbalance, or dehydration. It may also interact with certain medications or have adverse effects in individuals with certain health conditions. It's important to use cascara sagrada under the guidance of a healthcare professional and to discontinue use if any adverse effects occur.

Cell Food:

Definition: Cell Food is a dietary supplement marketed as a highly oxygenating and alkalizing formula. It's claimed to support overall health and vitality by providing essential nutrients and oxygen to the cells.

Ingredients: The exact ingredients of Cell Food can vary depending on the brand, but it typically contains a proprietary blend of minerals, enzymes, electrolytes, and trace elements. Some common ingredients may include purified water, dissolved oxygen, seawater extract, and plant-based enzymes.

How to Prepare: Cell Food is usually available in liquid form and is typically taken orally. It can be consumed directly or diluted in water or juice before consumption.

Dosage: The dosage of Cell Food can vary depending on the specific product and individual needs. It's important to follow the recommended dosage on the product label or consult with a healthcare professional for personalized guidance.

How to Use: Cell Food is typically taken orally, either directly or mixed into water or juice. It's important to shake the bottle well before use and to store it according to the manufacturer's instructions.

Side Effects: Cell Food is generally considered safe for most people when used as directed. However, some individuals may experience mild digestive upset or allergic reactions to certain ingredients. It's essential to consult with a healthcare provider before starting any new supplement regimen, especially if you have underlying health conditions or are taking medications.

Chaparral:

Definition: Chaparral, scientifically known as Larrea tridentata, is a shrub native to the southwestern United States and northern Mexico. It has been used for centuries by Native American tribes for its medicinal properties and is commonly used in herbal medicine today.

Ingredients: Chaparral contains several bioactive compounds, including nordihydroguaiaretic acid (NDGA), flavonoids, lignans, and volatile oils. NDGA is believed to be the primary active compound responsible for many of chaparral's therapeutic effects.

How to Prepare: Chaparral can be prepared and consumed in various forms, including teas, tinctures, capsules, and topical preparations. To make tea, dried chaparral leaves are steeped in hot water for several minutes before being strained and consumed. Tinctures are prepared by steeping the herb in alcohol or vinegar to extract its active compounds.

Dosage: The appropriate dosage of chaparral can vary depending on the specific form and intended use. It's important to follow the recommended dosage on the product label or consult with a healthcare professional for personalized guidance.

How to Use: Chaparral tea or tincture is typically taken orally. It can also be applied topically to the skin for certain conditions. It's important to use chaparral products as directed and to discontinue use if any adverse effects occur.

Side Effects: Chaparral is generally considered safe for most people when used in moderate amounts. However, excessive intake or prolonged use may lead to liver toxicity or other adverse effects. It may also interact with certain medications or have adverse effects in individuals with certain health conditions. It's important to use chaparral under the guidance of a healthcare professional and to discontinue use if any adverse effects occur.

Cocolmeca:

Definition: Cocolmeca, also known as Smilax ornata or sarsaparilla, is a flowering vine native to Mexico and Central America. It has been used traditionally in Mexican and Central American folk medicine for its purported medicinal properties.

Ingredients: Cocolmeca contains various bioactive compounds, including saponins, flavonoids, and plant sterols. These compounds are believed to contribute to the herb's medicinal properties, including its potential as a diuretic, blood purifier, and anti-inflammatory agent.

How to Prepare: Cocolmeca is commonly prepared and consumed as an herbal tea or decoction. To make tea, dried cocolmeca roots or leaves are steeped in hot water for several minutes before being strained and consumed. Decoctions involve boiling the roots or leaves in water to extract their active compounds.

Dosage: The appropriate dosage of cocolmeca can vary depending on factors such as age, health status, and the specific preparation being used. It's important to follow the recommended dosage on the product label or consult with a qualified herbalist or healthcare professional for personalized guidance.

How to Use: Cocolmeca tea or decoction is typically taken orally. It can also be used topically for certain skin conditions. It's important to use cocolmeca products as directed and to discontinue use if any adverse effects occur.

Side Effects: Cocolmeca is generally considered safe for most people when used in moderate amounts. However, excessive intake may lead to digestive upset or other adverse effects. It may also interact with certain medications or have adverse effects in individuals with certain health conditions. It's important to use cocolmeca under the guidance of a healthcare professional and to discontinue use if any adverse effects occur.

Contribo:

Definition: Contribo, also known as Aristolochiatrilobata, is a vine native to the Caribbean and Central America. It has been used traditionally in folk medicine for various purposes, including as a remedy for digestive issues, inflammation, and pain relief.

Ingredients: Contribo contains several bioactive compounds, including aristolochic acids, flavonoids, and alkaloids. These compounds are believed to contribute to the herb's medicinal properties, including its potential as an anti-inflammatory and analgesic agent.

How to Prepare: Contribo is typically prepared and consumed as an herbal tea or decoction. To make tea, dried contribo leaves or stems are steeped in hot water for several minutes before being strained and consumed. Decoctions involve boiling the leaves or stems in water to extract their active compounds.

Dosage: The appropriate dosage of contribo can vary depending on factors such as age, health status, and the specific preparation being used. It's important to follow the recommended dosage on the product label or consult with a qualified herbalist or healthcare professional for personalized guidance.

How to Use: Contribo tea or decoction is typically taken orally. It's important to use contribo products as directed and to discontinue use if any adverse effects occur.

Side Effects: Contribo contains aristolochic acids, which have been associated with serious adverse effects, including kidney damage and cancer. Due to these safety concerns, the use of contribo is highly discouraged, and it's important to avoid products containing aristolochic acids. Individuals should seek alternative remedies for their health needs.

Dandelion Root:

Definition: Dandelion, scientifically known as Taraxacum officinale, is a common flowering plant found worldwide. While often considered a pesky weed, dandelion has a long history of use in traditional medicine for its various health benefits.

Ingredients: Dandelion root contains several bioactive compounds, including sesquiterpene lactones, triterpenes, flavonoids, and polysaccharides. These compounds are believed to contribute to the herb's medicinal properties, including its potential as a diuretic, digestive aid, and liver tonic.

How to Prepare: Dandelion root can be prepared and consumed in various forms, including teas, tinctures, capsules, and extracts. To make tea, dried dandelion root is steeped in hot water for several minutes before being strained and consumed. Tinctures are prepared by steeping the root in alcohol or vinegar to extract its active compounds.

Dosage: The appropriate dosage of dandelion root can vary depending on factors such as age, health status, and the specific preparation being used. It's important to follow the recommended dosage on the product label or consult with a qualified herbalist or healthcare professional for personalized guidance.

How to Use: Dandelion root tea, tincture, or capsules are typically taken orally. It's important to use dandelion root products as directed and to discontinue use if any adverse effects occur.

Side Effects: Dandelion root is generally considered safe for most people when used in moderate amounts. However, some individuals may experience allergic reactions or digestive upset. It may also interact with certain medications or have adverse effects in individuals with certain health conditions. It's important to use dandelion root under the guidance of a healthcare professional and to discontinue use if any adverse effects occur.

Green Food Plus:

Definition: Green Food Plus is a dietary supplement formulated to provide a concentrated source of nutrients derived from various green plants. It's designed to support overall health and well-being by delivering essential vitamins, minerals, antioxidants, and phytonutrients.

Ingredients: Green Food Plus typically contains a blend of powdered green vegetables, grasses, algae, and other plant-based ingredients. Common ingredients may include wheatgrass, barley grass, spirulina, chlorella, alfalfa, kale, spinach, and broccoli, among others.

How to Prepare: Green Food Plus is usually available in powder form and can be mixed with water, juice, or smoothies. It's important to follow the recommended dosage on the product label and to consume it as part of a balanced diet.

Dosage: The appropriate dosage of Green Food Plus can vary depending on the specific product and individual needs. It's important to follow the recommended dosage on the product label or consult with a healthcare professional for personalized guidance.

How to Use: Green Food Plus powder is typically mixed with water, juice, or smoothies and consumed orally. It's often taken once or twice daily, preferably with meals, to maximize nutrient absorption.

Side Effects: Green Food Plus is generally considered safe for most people when used as directed. However, some individuals may experience digestive upset or allergic reactions to certain ingredients. It's important to consult with a healthcare provider before starting any new supplement regimen, especially if you have underlying health conditions or are taking medications.

Guaco:

Definition: Guaco, also known as Mikania cordata or Mikania glomerata, is a medicinal plant native to Central and South America. It has a long history of use in traditional medicine for its potential therapeutic properties.

Ingredients: Guaco contains several bioactive compounds, including coumarins, flavonoids, tannins, and saponins. These compounds are believed to contribute to the herb's medicinal properties, including its potential as an expectorant, anti-inflammatory, and antispasmodic agent.

How to Prepare: Guaco is typically prepared and consumed as an herbal tea or infusion. To make tea, dried guaco leaves are steeped in hot water for several minutes before being strained and consumed.

Dosage: The appropriate dosage of guaco can vary depending on factors such as age, health status, and the specific preparation being used. It's important to follow the recommended dosage on the product label or consult with a qualified herbalist or healthcare professional for personalized guidance.

How to Use: Guaco tea is typically taken orally. It can be consumed on its own or mixed with honey or other herbal teas for added flavor.

Side Effects: Guaco is generally considered safe for most people when used in moderate amounts. However, some individuals may experience allergic reactions or digestive upset. It may also interact with certain medications or have adverse effects in individuals with certain health conditions. It's important to use guaco under the guidance of a healthcare professional and to discontinue use if any adverse effects occur.

Herban Iron:

Definition: Herban Iron is a dietary supplement designed to provide an easily absorbable form of iron to support healthy iron levels in the body. It's particularly beneficial for individuals with iron deficiency or anemia.

Ingredients: Herban Iron typically contains iron in the form of ferrous bisglycinate, which is a highly bioavailable and gentle form of iron that is less likely to cause digestive upset or constipation compared to other forms of iron. It may also contain other ingredients such as vitamin C to enhance iron absorption.

How to Prepare: Herban Iron is usually available in capsule or liquid form. Capsules are taken orally with water, while liquid forms may be mixed with water or juice before consumption. It's important to follow the recommended dosage on the product label.

Dosage: The appropriate dosage of Herban Iron depends on factors such as age, gender, and the severity of iron deficiency. It's important to consult with a healthcare professional to determine the correct dosage for individual needs.

How to Use: Herban Iron capsules are typically taken orally with water, while liquid forms may be mixed with water or juice before consumption. It's important to take Herban Iron as directed and to avoid taking it with dairy products, antacids, or other substances that may interfere with iron absorption.

Side Effects: While Herban Iron is generally considered safe for most people when used as directed, some individuals may experience mild side effects such as gastrointestinal discomfort or constipation. It's important to consult with a healthcare professional before starting any new supplement regimen, especially if you have underlying health conditions or are taking medications.

Hydrangea:

Definition: Hydrangea, scientifically known as Hydrangea arborescens, is a flowering shrub native to North America. It has been used traditionally in herbal medicine for its potential diuretic and anti-inflammatory properties.

Ingredients: Hydrangea contains several bioactive compounds, including saponins, flavonoids, and glycosides. These compounds are believed to contribute to the herb's medicinal properties, including its potential as a diuretic, kidney tonic, and anti-inflammatory agent.

How to Prepare: Hydrangea root is typically prepared and consumed as an herbal tea or tincture. To make tea, dried hydrangea root is steeped in hot water for several minutes before being strained and consumed. Tinctures are prepared by steeping the root in alcohol or vinegar to extract its active compounds.

Dosage: The appropriate dosage of hydrangea can vary depending on factors such as age, health status, and the specific preparation being used. It's important to follow the recommended dosage on the product label or consult with a qualified herbalist or healthcare professional for personalized guidance.

How to Use: Hydrangea tea or tincture is typically taken orally. It's important to use hydrangea products as directed and to discontinue use if any adverse effects occur.

Side Effects: Hydrangea is generally considered safe for most people when used in moderate amounts. However, some individuals may experience digestive upset or allergic reactions. It may also interact with certain medications or have adverse effects in individuals with certain health conditions. It's important to use hydrangea under the guidance of a healthcare professional and to discontinue use if any adverse effects occur.

Irish Moss:

Definition: Irish Moss, scientifically known as Chondrus crispus, is a species of red algae or seaweed native to the Atlantic coastlines of Europe and North America. It has been used for centuries in traditional Irish and Scottish cuisine, as well as in herbal medicine.

Ingredients: Irish Moss is rich in various nutrients, including iodine, sulfur compounds, vitamins (such as vitamin A, vitamin K, and vitamin B12), minerals (including calcium, magnesium, potassium, and sodium), and polysaccharides (such as carrageenan). These nutrients are believed to contribute to the herb's potential health benefits.

How to Prepare: Irish Moss is typically prepared by soaking it in water to rehydrate and soften it before use. It can be added to soups, stews, smoothies, desserts, and other dishes as a thickening agent or nutritional supplement.

Dosage: The appropriate dosage of Irish Moss can vary depending on factors such as age, health status, and the specific preparation being used. It's important to follow recipes or guidelines for culinary use and to consult with a healthcare professional for guidance on using Irish Moss as a dietary supplement.

How to Use: Irish Moss can be used in culinary applications to add thickness and nutritional value to dishes. It can also be consumed as a dietary supplement in the form of capsules, powders, or extracts.

Side Effects: Irish Moss is generally considered safe for most people when consumed in moderate amounts as part of a balanced diet. However, some individuals may be allergic to seaweed or carrageenan, a compound found in Irish Moss that is used as a food additive. It's important to discontinue use if any adverse effects occur and to consult with a healthcare professional if you have any concerns.

Irish Sea Moss:

Definition: Irish Sea Moss is a term often used interchangeably with Irish Moss, referring to the same species of red algae, Chondrus crispus. It's harvested from the rocky shores of the Atlantic coastlines of Europe and North America.

Ingredients: Irish Sea Moss shares the same nutritional profile as Irish Moss, containing iodine, vitamins, minerals, and polysaccharides. It's valued for its potential health benefits, including supporting thyroid function, boosting immune health, and promoting digestion.

How to Prepare: Irish Sea Moss is prepared in the same way as Irish Moss, by soaking it in water to rehydrate and soften it before use. It can be used in culinary applications or consumed as a dietary supplement.

Dosage: The dosage of Irish Sea Moss depends on the form and intended use. As a dietary supplement, it's important to follow the recommended dosage on the product label or consult with a healthcare professional for personalized guidance.

How to Use: Irish Sea Moss can be used in various culinary applications, including soups, smoothies, desserts, and sauces. It can also be consumed as a dietary supplement in the form of capsules, powders, or extracts.

Side Effects: Similar to Irish Moss, Irish Sea Moss is generally considered safe for most people when consumed in moderate amounts. However, individuals with seaweed allergies or sensitivities to carrageenan should exercise caution. It's important to discontinue use if any adverse effects occur and to consult with a healthcare professional if you have any concerns.

Lymphalin:

Definition: Lymphalin is a herbal supplement formulated to support lymphatic system health. The lymphatic system plays a crucial role in immune function and waste removal in the body, and Lymphalin is designed to promote its proper function.

Ingredients: Lymphalin typically contains a blend of herbs and botanical extracts known for their traditional use in supporting lymphatic system health. Common ingredients may include cleavers, red clover, echinacea, burdock root, and calendula, among others.

How to Prepare: Lymphalin is usually available in capsule or liquid form. Capsules are taken orally with water, while liquid forms may be mixed with water or juice before consumption. It's important to follow the recommended dosage on the product label.

Dosage: The appropriate dosage of Lymphalin can vary depending on the specific product and individual needs. It's important to follow the recommended dosage on the product label or consult with a healthcare professional for personalized guidance.

How to Use: Lymphalin capsules are typically taken orally with water, while liquid forms may be mixed with water or juice before consumption. It's often recommended to take Lymphalin on an empty stomach for optimal absorption.

Side Effects: Lymphalin is generally considered safe for most people when used as directed. However, some individuals may experience mild side effects such as gastrointestinal discomfort or allergic reactions to certain ingredients. It's important to consult with a healthcare provider before starting any new supplement regimen, especially if you have underlying health conditions or are taking medications.

Manjakani:

Definition: Manjakani, also known as Quercus infectoria or oak gall, is a natural substance derived from the oak tree. It has been used for centuries in traditional medicine for its potential health benefits, particularly for women's health and vaginal tightening.

Ingredients: Manjakani contains various bioactive compounds, including tannins, flavonoids, and gallic acid. These compounds are believed to contribute to the herb's medicinal properties, including its potential as an astringent and antiseptic agent.

How to Prepare: Manjakani is typically available in powder, capsule, or liquid extract form. It can be taken orally or used topically depending on the intended use. For vaginal tightening, manjakani may be applied topically as a gel or inserted into the vagina in capsule form.

Dosage: The appropriate dosage of manjakani can vary depending on factors such as age, health status, and the specific preparation being used. It's important to follow the recommended dosage on the product label or consult with a qualified herbalist or healthcare professional for personalized guidance.

How to Use: Manjakani can be taken orally or used topically depending on the intended use. It's important to use manjakani products as directed and to discontinue use if any adverse effects occur.

Side Effects: Manjakani is generally considered safe for most people when used in moderate amounts. However, some individuals may experience allergic reactions or skin irritation when used topically. It's important to use manjakani under the guidance of a healthcare professional and to discontinue use if any adverse effects occur.

Red Clover:

Definition: Red clover, scientifically known as Trifolium pratense, is a flowering plant belonging to the legume family. It's native to Europe, Western Asia, and Northwest Africa but has been naturalized in many other regions. Red clover has been used in traditional medicine for various purposes, including its potential to support women's health and menopausal symptoms.

Ingredients: Red clover contains several bioactive compounds, including isoflavones (such as genistein and daidzein), flavonoids, and phytoestrogens. These compounds are believed to contribute to the herb's medicinal properties, including its potential as a hormone-balancing agent and its ability to support cardiovascular health.

How to Prepare: Red clover is typically prepared and consumed as an herbal tea or tincture. To make tea, dried red clover flowers are steeped in hot water for several minutes before being strained and consumed. Tinctures are prepared by steeping the flowers in alcohol or vinegar to extract their active compounds.

Dosage: The appropriate dosage of red clover can vary depending on factors such as age, health status, and the specific preparation being used. It's important to follow the recommended dosage on the product label or consult with a qualified herbalist or healthcare professional for personalized guidance.

How to Use: Red clover tea or tincture is typically taken orally. It's important to use red clover products as directed and to discontinue use if any adverse effects occur.

Side Effects: Red clover is generally considered safe for most people when used in moderate amounts. However, some individuals may experience allergic reactions or digestive upset. It may also interact with certain medications or have adverse effects in individuals with certain health conditions. It's important to use red clover under the guidance of a healthcare professional and to discontinue use if any adverse effects occur.

Red Raspberry:

Definition: Red raspberry, scientifically known as Rubus idaeus, is a species of raspberry native to Europe and northern Asia. It's widely cultivated for its delicious berries and has been used in traditional medicine for various purposes, including its potential to support women's health during pregnancy and childbirth.

Ingredients: Red raspberry contains several bioactive compounds, including flavonoids, ellagic acid, anthocyanins, and vitamin C. These compounds are believed to contribute to the herb's medicinal properties, including its potential as an antioxidant, anti-inflammatory, and uterine tonic.

How to Prepare: Red raspberry leaf is typically prepared and consumed as an herbal tea or infusion. To make tea, dried red raspberry leaves are steeped in hot water for several minutes before being strained and consumed.

Dosage: The appropriate dosage of red raspberry leaf can vary depending on factors such as age, health status, and the specific preparation being used. It's important to follow the recommended dosage on the product label or consult with a qualified herbalist or healthcare professional for personalized guidance.

How to Use: Red raspberry leaf tea is typically taken orally. It's often recommended for pregnant individuals in the later stages of pregnancy to support uterine health and prepare for childbirth. It's important to use red raspberry leaf products as directed and to discontinue use if any adverse effects occur.

Side Effects: Red raspberry leaf is generally considered safe for most people when used in moderate amounts. However, some individuals may experience allergic reactions or digestive upset. Pregnant individuals should consult with a healthcare professional before using red raspberry leaf, especially if they have any underlying health conditions or are taking medications. It's important to use red raspberry leaf under the guidance of a healthcare professional and to discontinue use if any adverse effects occur.

Rhubarb:

Definition: Rhubarb, scientifically known as Rheum rhabarbarum, is a perennial plant cultivated for its edible stalks. While primarily used in culinary applications, rhubarb has also been utilized in traditional medicine for its potential health benefits, particularly for digestive health.

Ingredients: Rhubarb stalks contain various bioactive compounds, including anthraquinones (such as emodin and rhein), fiber, vitamins (such as vitamin K), and minerals (including calcium and potassium). These compounds are believed to contribute to the herb's medicinal properties, including its potential as a laxative and digestive aid.

How to Prepare: Rhubarb stalks are typically cooked before consumption, as the raw stalks are very tart and can be unpleasant to eat. They are often used in pies, crisps, jams, sauces, and other desserts, as well as in savory dishes. Rhubarb can also be used to make compotes, jams, and preserves.

Dosage: There is no specific dosage for rhubarb in culinary applications, as it is used as a food rather than a medicinal herb. However, when used for its potential laxative effects, it's important to consume rhubarb in moderation to avoid gastrointestinal upset.

How to Use: Rhubarb stalks can be chopped and cooked in various dishes, including pies, sauces, and jams. It's important to remove and discard the leaves, as they contain toxic compounds. When using rhubarb for its potential laxative effects, it's typically consumed as part of a cooked dish or in the form of a rhubarb-based herbal remedy.

Side Effects: Rhubarb stalks are generally safe for most people when consumed in moderate amounts as part of a balanced diet. However, excessive intake may lead to digestive upset or adverse effects due to the presence of oxalic acid, which can bind to calcium and form kidney stones in susceptible individuals. It's important to use rhubarb in moderation and to consult with a healthcare professional if you have any concerns or underlying health conditions.

THE END